How To Quit Smoking For Good

312 Effective Tips To Stop Smoking Cigarettes

ADAM COLTON

Published by BizMove
www.bizmove.com

ISBN: 1979528659
ISBN- 978-1979528658

312 Effective Tips To Stop Smoking Cigarettes

Most smokers admit that they would like to quit and wish they had never started smoking in the first place. Most have also previously tried to quit to no avail. But you can try again and with the help of the following tips and tricks, you can become a proud non-smoker.

1. If you're trying to quit smoking, try chewing gum instead. Often times when you try to leave a bad habit behind, you must replace it with a more positive one. Chewing gum allows you to use your mouth and jaw in some of the same ways that smoking does. It is a healthy way to keep yourself busy while you're working toward quitting.

2. Sometimes people think they can quit smoking by switching to a product such as chewing-tobacco. This isn't a good idea because usually chewing-tobacco contains more nicotine. You might end up just replacing one addiction for another. If you really want a product that can help you quit, try nicotine gum instead. You can slowly taper off the gum. They don't usually sell progressively weaker versions of chewing tobacco.

3. Make sure you get lots of rest if you are quitting smoking. Lots of people find that if they stay up

late, they are more inclined to crave cigarettes. Additionally, you will be alone late at night, increasing your temptation to smoke. Getting plenty of sleep will not only limit the time you sit around thinking about cigarettes, it will also help your body to overcome nicotine withdrawal.

4. To keep yourself motivated to quit smoking, be clear about why you want to quit. While there are many good reasons to quit smoking, you want to focus on your most powerful, personal reasons. Every time you feel tempted, remind yourself how much you want to improve your health, save money or set a good example for your kids.

5. Talk to your doctor about prescription medicines. If you want to ease nicotine withdrawal symptoms, consider prescription medications. There are certain medications that affect the chemical balance in your brain and can help reduce cravings. There are also drugs that can reduce bothersome withdrawal symptoms, like inability to concentrate or depression.

6. When quitting smoking, you must learn to manage your stress. Once smoking is no longer an option, turn to healthier outlets such as massage therapy, long walks in your favorite park, listening to relaxing music, or meditation. Find something you

can do that provides near-instant gratification so that you'll be less tempted to turn to smoking when things get tough.

7. Switching the band of cigarette you smoke can help lead you to quitting. Consider smoking a brand you don't like. Don´t smoke more than normal or in a different way. This will get you started on your way to stop smoking.

8. Many smokers have certain triggers that create the sudden need for a cigarette, such as feeling stressed, ending a meal, or being at a certain location. When you are trying to quit, avoid these triggers if you can. If you can't avoid them, come up with some way to distract yourself from the need to smoke.

9. Find out specifics on how quitting smoking will improve your health. There are many statistics out there about how dramatically different your odds of contracting diseases are if you don't smoke. Find out too how soon you can expect to experience other small perks like improved breathing and sense of taste.

10.   Write down a journal of every time you have a cigarette and what your reasons were for having one. This journal will help you to find out what your smoking triggers are. For some it may be the

first morning cigarette, or the need to smoke after a meal. For others, it may be stress. Determining your triggers will help you to figure out a way to fight them.

11.	To make quitting smoking seem more straightforward, put the negatives of your smoking habit into numbers. For example, figure out how often you smoke, how many cigarettes you smoke a day and how much it costs you to smoke that much on a daily, monthly and yearly basis. Every time you cut back a little, you'll know exactly how much you've progressed.

12.	If you can do away with things that remind you of smoking, it will be easier to resist temptation. Things you should eliminate includes removing ashtrays and cigarette lighters. To get rid of smoke odors in your home, clean your house and wash your clothes. Taking these steps can reduce your urges to smoke a cigarette because you are removing potential triggers.

13.	Remind yourself of how gross cigarettes are. This will help you focus on quitting because you will think about how dirty they are. Avoid emptying ashtrays so you can see how much you've smoked and the terrible smell it leaves behind. You may also want to try filling a jar with the butts and ashes as a reminder.

14.   Start exercising! If you are active it can help to reduce symptoms of withdrawal and nicotine cravings. Rather than reaching for a cigarette, get off the couch and exercise, or go for a walk. This will really help to take off your mind of smoking, and is also a great way to improve your physical fitness.

15.   Positive thinking makes a big difference when it comes to quitting smoking. You will be able to better conquer temptations if you recognize every day without smoking, as an achievement in itself. By keeping track of small goals, you can keep your self-esteem high and hopefully, conquer that habit for good!

16.   You need to eat a balanced diet. Do not quit smoking and start a diet in the same week. Follow a healthy, balanced diet. If you smoke, veggies and fruit can give a bad mouth taste if you smoke. If you eat these items when you do not smoke, you will be doing a huge favor to your health, and it will help you stay away from those harmful cigarettes.

17.   If you want to quit smoking, the word for you is "No". Every time you're tempted you have to

disallow yourself the ability to say "Yes" to a cigarette. If your only answer is "No" you'll find that you can't cave in to a craving. No cigarettes, no "Maybe", leads to no smoking!

18.   If you're doing well on your stop smoking journey, don't forget to reward yourself. Treat yourself to a nice massage, a pedicure, or a special new outfit when you've cut back, and then something else when you've stopped entirely. You need to have rewards like this to look forward to, as they can help to keep you motivated.

19.   Deal with nicotine withdrawal. Once you quit smoking, nicotine withdrawal can make you anxious, frustrated, or depressed. It's all too easy to revert to your old habit. Nicotine replacement therapy can really help to relieve these symptoms. Whether it's in the form of gum, a patch, or a lozenge, using one of these will probably double your chances of succeeding.

20.   Make sure you do not feel as if you have to give up any aspect of your life because you are quitting smoking. Anything that you do you can still do as an ex-smoker. Who knows, you may even be able to do your favorite things a little bit better.

21.   If you're a smoker who lights up more in social situations, plan ways to not join your friends for a cigarette when you're out. While dining, stay at the table if your friends go outside for to smoke. If you're at a party, if people are smoking, find a non-smoker to chat with. Finding ways to not be around smokers will make it easier for you to quit.

22.   The most important thing to do when you want to stop smoking is to make that initial commitment to the change. Instead of setting a deadline that you can keep pushing back, quit today. Just stop smoking and do not ever start again. This technique may be tough, but the benefits are extraordinary. In the long-term, the method is the successful one.

23.   Write down why you're quitting ahead of time and keep that list handy. When that craving hits you, refer to your list for motivation. Understanding ahead of time why quitting is important to you will help to keep you focused in those moments of weakness, and it might even help to get you back on track if you should slip up.

24.   Don't assume that a nicotine withdrawal medication has to have nicotine in it. While it is true that you can find an alternate source of nicotine and reduce your levels of it, you could just try a prescription medication that blocks your need for

nicotine. Consult your physician about a medicine that might just kill your cravings.

25.   Start moving. Physical activity is a great for reducing nicotine cravings and can ease some of the withdrawal symptoms. When you crave a cigarette, go for a jog instead. Even mild exercise can be helpful, like pulling the weeds in the garden or taking a leisurely stroll. Plus, the extra activity will burn extra calories and help ward off any weight gain as you are quitting smoking.

26.   You can replace your smoking habit with positive coping habits instead. This means really looking inside yourself and examining your habits. If you smoke when you are stressed out, consider how you can diffuse the negative energy instead. Some people find solace in meditative and deep breathing exercises, but you can experiment with a variety of techniques to find one that suits you.

27.   If you want to quit smoking, stop buying cigarettes. It kind of goes without saying that if you don't have cigarettes on you, it will be much more difficult to smoke. Throw away any cigarettes that are currently in your possession and make a pact with yourself not to buy any more.

28.   To make quitting smoking seem more straightforward, put the negatives of your smoking habit into numbers. For example, figure out how often you smoke, how many cigarettes you smoke a day and how much it costs you to smoke that much on a daily, monthly and yearly basis. Every time you cut back a little, you'll know exactly how much you've progressed.

29.   Do not try to start smoking without first developing a plan. Your life has probably been ruled by cigarettes for quite some time. A life without cigarettes will require adjustments in your life. Deciding what you are going to do about cravings, avoiding triggers, and setting your quit date are all essential components of a successful plan for quitting.

30.   Exercising can help replace your smoking habit. Your brain releases endorphins after you work out, which will improve your mood. A workout is also an excellent distraction from your cravings. Exercise will also help boost your metabolism to make up for the hit it takes when you quit smoking, reducing your potential weight gain.

31.   While you are in the process of quitting smoking, consume vegetables, fruits, seeds and nuts. Eating a healthy, well-balanced diet of natural

foods can help for many reasons. First, you can behaviorally replace smoking motions by keeping you r mouth and hands occupied. Also, your chances of gaining weight during this quit period is reduced. The vitamins and other nutrients can also improve the way you feel while going through withdrawals.

32.   If you're trying to quit smoking, stopping "cold turkey" is a bad idea. Quitting without a means of support for nicotine withdrawal is an uphill battle. Because nicotine is addictive, it's very easy to relapse without some form of support when quitting. It's best to use smoking cessation medicine, or some type of therapy when you're ready to quit.

33.   To keep your hands and mouth busy while trying to quit smoking, keep crunchy vegetables like carrots or celery on hand. These low-calorie snacks will not only keep your hands busy, but they will steady your blood sugar and keep you from reaching for higher-calorie foods that could lead to weight gain.

34.   Though aversion therapies have gotten a bad rap recently, they do sometimes work in helping you to stop smoking. They do not need to be extravagant methods and you don't need to pay a therapist to

employ aversion techniques. Try the simple things, such as permeating your favorite sweater with the smoke from that last cigarette you smoke. Then reach for it after not smoking for a day or two; you will be appalled at the offensive odor that you have been subjecting yourself and others to on a daily basis.

35.   It is extremely important that you talk to a doctor prior to quitting smoking. This person can provide you some advice on your best methods of quitting. In addition, he or she can provide you some additional support on your journey. Both of these things greatly increase your chances of quitting for good.

36.   The health of your loved ones depends on you to quit smoking. Smoking is harmful for you and anyone around you that inhales secondhand smoke, and people can even get cancer from it. If you stop smoking, you are removing secondhand smoke from your loved ones lives. Not only will you be healthier when you stop smoking, but your loved ones will also be healthier, too.

37.   To improve your odds of quitting smoking for good, don't combine your effort to quit with another goal, particularly weight loss. You already have enough stress and cravings to deal with just

trying to quit smoking. If you try to wean yourself from something else at the same time, you are likely to fail at both.

38.   As you begin your journey to a smoke free lifestyle, plan a series of rewards as you reach certain milestones. Make a list of the rewards you will offer yourself once you've stopped smoking for one day, a week, a month and so on. Put this list on the refrigerator and look at it every morning before work or school. This might just help to keep you motivated during times of weakness.

39.   Make sure you tell yourself that you are not going to smoke each and every day. As you get up in the morning, you should try telling yourself that you are not going to smoke a single cigarette. Reaffirming this goal in your mind each morning will keep you on track to successful smoking cessation.

40.   Take the time and money you save by quitting smoking, and apply it to exercising. Mood boosting endorphins are released with exercise and you will be distracted from your cravings by physical activity. Exercise can also help avoid possible weight gain caused by the changes nicotine withdrawal can make to your metabolism.

41.   Throw away your cigarettes and lighters. This will make it impossible to smoke unless you leave the house. It serves to remind you how much of a hassle it is to smoke and leaves you without any. When you do this, keep yourself busy with other activities so you don't think about smoking.

42.   If you are pregnant, or plan or becoming that way, then use this as a serious motivation to stop smoking. Statistics say that women who smoke while carrying a child, especially in the first trimester, will cause the infant to have a decreased body weight. This will in turn affect their health, potentially throughout childhood.

43.   In order to quit, you must believe that you can do it. While the physical cravings and withdrawal symptoms of smoking are difficult, your brain is the most important item in your fight. You must be able to work past your cravings and that fight is all mental. Believe that you can do it and you will see success.

44.   Follow a smart diet. Now is not the time to diet! Just focus on making health food choices. Studies show that smokers receive a poor taste in their mouth from fruits and vegetables as well as low-fat dairy products. Eating these types of food will not

only boost your health but also help you quit smoking.

45.   To assist in your quest to ban smoking from your life, seek out another smoker who is attempting to quit, and provide each other some support. The only people who can truly understand what you're going through are the ones who are going through the exact same situation you are in. Share tips with each other and give positive words to each other, whenever one of you feels like giving in to temptation. Trying to quit with someone else is much more effective than trying to quit on your own.

46.   When you quit smoking, don't forget to drink plenty of water. Drinking water has beneficial effects anyway, but especially when you're trying to stop smoking. It will help flush out the toxins that smoking leaves behind, as well as help satiate your oral fixation, if you have one. If you already drink plenty of water, think about drinking an extra glass the next time you have a craving for a cigarette.

47.   In order to quit smoking successfully, ask for help from the people you see most. Having the support of family, friends, and co-workers can mean the difference between success and failure. Quitting any habit is difficult, especially one like

smoking that is addictive. Make sure the people around you cheer you on and do not intentionally thwart your success.

48.   When aiming to kick the smoking habit for good, you should always believe that you can do it. Think about all the incredible things you have accomplished in your life so far. This will help you realize you have the strength to overcome this addiction. Having faith in yourself is not only important for quitting smoking, but it's also important for overall success in your life.

49.   You must know why you want to stop smoking. Having shallow reasons, like it is bad for you are not good enough. To really get yourself motivated, you need a personal and powerful reason to quit. Maybe you are scared of lung cancer. Or maybe you would like to keep your family from second hand smoke. It might be because you want to both feel and look younger. Choose a strong reason that outweighs your urge to light up.

50.   Ensure that you're getting an adequate amount of sleep when you're in the process of giving up your smoking habit. Lots of people find that if they stay up late, they are more inclined to crave cigarettes. Many times, there is nobody around during late night hours, which makes it easier to

sneak in a couple puffs. If you get eight hours of sleep every night, you will be able to focus better, which means you can control cravings better.

51.   Don't Go Cold Turkey

52.   Do not quit cold turkey. It can be tempting to throw out your cigarettes and say, "I quit!" But cold turkey is not the way you want to go. Studies show that over ninety percent of people who try to quit smoking with no medication or therapy end up relapsing. The reason for this is because nicotine is addictive and your brain craves it. Without it, nicotine withdrawal symptoms set in.

53.   Try not to eat too much to fill the void left from quitting cigarettes. Nicotine is an appetite suppressant, so do not be surprised when you start to feel hungrier after quitting. Eat healthier when you quit smoking cigarettes. This will give you more room for calories you will consume by snacking.

54.   To quit smoking for good, you'll get better results by gradually weaning yourself than you would if you tried to quit cold turkey. Nearly all people that try to quit cold turkey fail as a result of nicotine withdrawal. Cut back slowly and steadily, and if the cravings are still too powerful then

subsidize your efforts with medication or other tools.

55.   If you find it too daunting to quit smoking cold-turkey, consider helping the process along by trying replacements like nicotine patches or gum. These are found over the counter at any pharmacy and give your body a small amount of nicotine, which can lessen withdrawal symptoms and get you through the worst times.

56.   If you have very strong associations between smoking and drinking coffee or smoking while you're drinking, you may need to avoid these triggers for a while. Once you feel comfortable enough in your ability to stay away from cigarettes, you can slowly bring back that morning cup of joe or happy hour with your friends.

57.   Blow off some steam to keep yourself from blowing smoke. One of the most effective ways for you to work through nicotine cravings is to exercise. As an added bonus, you will feel the effects of your improving health more readily if you subsidize quitting smoking with a more rigorous exercise routine.

58.   Join a support group to help you in your quest to quit smoking. A support group can commiserate

with you about the difficulties that quitting smoking entails, and share their coping mechanisms. The leader of the group may also be able to teach you behavior modification techniques, or other strategies that can prove helpful.

59.   When trying to quit smoking, set a goal. Tell yourself that you want to quit by a certain date and that if you are successful, you will reward yourself with something you have been wanting. You can use the money you saved by not smoking to buy this treat! This will give you the motivation you need.

60.   Use visualization in order to assist you in quitting your smoking habit. When doing deep breathing exercises, shut your eyes, and imagine yourself being a non-smoker. Imagine yourself not giving in to temptation. Imagine winning a medal for not smoking. These types of programs, referred to as "quit smoking hypnosis," are extremely effective.

61.   Your family and loved ones offer the greatest motivation for quitting. They can be affected by not only your possible illness or death, but also by negative health consequences from being around your smoke. Statistics say that one in five deaths in

America alone are tied to smoking cigarettes. Do not become a statistic.

62.   Exercise can replace smoking. You'll get an endorphin boost that will keep you from worrying as much about cigarettes. Exercise also helps to compensate for your metabolism slowing down as you quit, which will help you minimize the weight gain you experience.

63.   You will find it hard to do some of your normal routines while you are quitting smoking. For example, going to a bar with friends who smoke. When your friend goes outside for a cigarette, resist the urge to go with them to keep them company. Everything that you once did as a smoker, you will be able to do again.

64.   Remember that smoking cessation is really all about replacing one behavior with another. For most people, it is primarily the physical act of smoking that is the major draw. It signifies "me time" and a break from a hectic schedule or a boring job. Choose ahead of time exactly what behavior you will replace those smoking minutes with, and then do it!

65.   If you're trying to quit smoking, try quitting cold turkey. This method is the easiest in the long run.

While this may seem a lot more difficult when you are starting out, it is much easier than stringing your self along. Be honest with your self and commit to the quit and you will be off cigarettes fairly easily.

66.   If decide to give up smoking, try hypnosis. Seeing a licensed hypnotist can be effective and has proven successful for many people. During hypnosis, the hypnotist will give you positive affirmations while you are hypnotized. This hypnosis will tell your brain that smoking is not appealing, helping you avoid the urge to smoke.

67.   It does not matter how long it has been since you gave up smoking, you can never have "just one". You are a nicotine addict. While just one does not mean you will be smoking a packet a day again by morning, it will mean that you have "just one more" a lot sooner than you would like.

68.   Find healthy stress relief methods to help deal with your nicotine cravings and withdrawal. Get some exercise when cravings hit, engage in a hobby or teach your partner to give a great massage. When you have downtime, surround yourself with pleasant distractions, such as good books, scheduled chats with friends or new games.

69.   When you are trying to quit smoking, be sure that you are drinking plenty of water. Not only is water good for you, but it also fulfills the need to have something in your mouth. Also, large amounts of water help to clear out nicotine and other chemicals in your body caused by cigarettes.

70.   Always keep in mind that there is only one outcome from taking another puff of a cigarette. That outcome is smoking again at the level that you were at, until the habit cripples you and you are in the hospital dying. This is a scary truth that will help you stay on track.

71.   Realize that you will experience times of stress, so make a specific plan for countering this. Most people who smoke will light up when they're stressed out. If you make a plan and have strategies in place, you can better avoid smoking. Keep a back-up plan handy in case plan A doesn't work out.

72.   Find out specifics on how quitting smoking will improve your health. There are many statistics out there about how dramatically different your odds of contracting diseases are if you don't smoke. Find out too how soon you can expect to experience other small perks like improved breathing and sense of taste.

73.   You'll be more successful in your attempt to quit smoking if you ease down on how many cigarettes you smoke per day. You can create a set schedule for when you can smoke, and how many cigarettes per day you'll smoke, gradually letting yourself smoke fewer and fewer until a set date when you'll completely stop.

74.   Consider joining a support group when you decide to stop smoking. If your schedule does not allow for regular meetings, then look for telephone help lines or ones where people can log in online. These groups will give you instant access to support, regardless of what time you need them.

75.   If you decide to use a specific, dedicate program to help you stop smoking, remember that the more intense ones will have a much higher chance of success. This is not something that you can approach with a half-hearted effort. Counseling sessions or group therapy should be consistent, lasting at least 30 minutes and over a period of two weeks minimum.

76.   To assist in your quest to ban smoking from your life, seek out another smoker who is attempting to quit, and provide each other some support. The only people who can truly understand

what you're going through are the ones who are going through the exact same situation you are in. Share tips with each other and give positive words to each other, whenever one of you feels like giving in to temptation. Trying to quit with someone else is much more effective than trying to quit on your own.

77.   If you want to avoid nicotine withdrawals, but aren't comfortable using a nicotine replacement, talk to your doctor about medication. There are many prescription pills that help your body fight off cravings without giving it nicotine. These pills can also help you avoid some of the side effects of quitting smoking, like depression.

78.   To help you continue to stop smoking in the few days after you quit, you should avoid drinking beverages that you associate with smoking. Caffeine for instance, as many smokers are usually coffee drinkers. By avoiding these smoking triggers and replacing it with something you normally don't do while smoking, this can help you to remain smoke-free.

79.   If you are trying to quit smoking all together then you need to commit and stop carrying your cigarettes around with you. If you do not have cigarettes with you then you make it less convenient

to smoke. This will make it easier for you to quit in the long run.

80.   You must know why you want to stop smoking. Having shallow reasons, like it is bad for you are not good enough. To really get yourself motivated, you need a personal and powerful reason to quit. Maybe you are scared of lung cancer. Or maybe you would like to keep your family from second hand smoke. It might be because you want to both feel and look younger. Choose a strong reason that outweighs your urge to light up.

81.   Find another way to relax. Nicotine is a relaxant, so you need to find a substitute to lessen your stress. A massage or yoga is a really great way of relaxing, or you could try a warm bath, or listening to your favorite music. Whenever possible, try to stay away from anything stressful during the initial couple of weeks when you stop smoking.

82.   Once you commit to quitting smoking, give your home, car and other personal spaces and effects a thorough cleaning. Smelling smoke will only make you want to smoke. Likewise, your sense of smell will improve the longer you go without smoking, and cleaning will give you a chance to appreciate just how bad the smoke made your items smell.

83.   When you are fighting the urge to smoke, go and do some exercise. Not only will your body benefit while you are keeping fit, the physical activity can help to keep the urges at bay. Anything that can be used as a distraction while you are working through the crave is a great tool to use.

84.   Avoid triggering that make you want to smoke. Alcohol is a trigger for many, so when you are quitting, try to drink less. If coffee is your trigger, for a couple of weeks drink tea instead. If you like to smoke after eating a meal, do something else rather like taking a walk or brushing your teeth.

85.   When you're ready to quit smoking, and have a plan in place to do so, set a firm date after which you won't smoke anymore. Prepare for the date, and make a big deal out of it. Think of it as the day when you regain control of your life, and make it a joyous occasion.

86.   The best way to quit for good is to quit for the right reasons. You should not quit for the people around you. You should quit for yourself. You should make a decision that you want to live a happier, healthier lifestyle and stick to it. This is the best way to ensure success.

87. Remember the following acronym forever: N.O.P.E. It stands for "never one puff, ever." This will be a lifelong motto for you to follow, and it should be your mantra when you are tempted to have "just that one" cigarette. Even if you are out drinking with friends, remember to say N.O.P.E. to that puff!

88. Avoid emptying your ashtrays. If you see how many cigarettes you have smoked laying the the ashtray, you will be less likely to smoke any more. This will also leave the unsightly butts and their smell behind. This can be helpful because it will remind of you how bad the smell of smoke is.

89. Learn and use positive mantras. Tell yourself that you're strong and powerful and that you can quit. Let yourself know that you believe in yourself and that you know you will be successful. When you make positive mantras such as these, a part of your life, success will follow. This is as true for quitting smoking as it is for every other aspect of your life.

90. Start exercising! If you are active it can help to reduce symptoms of withdrawal and nicotine cravings. Rather than reaching for a cigarette, get off the couch and exercise, or go for a walk. This will really help to take off your mind of smoking,

and is also a great way to improve your physical fitness.

91.   Keep your hands and mouth busy when you are quitting smoking by eating lots of fruits and veggies. You are going to be in the habit of holding something in your hand and putting something in your mouth after years of smoking. If you keep these healthy snacks handy, you can reach for them instead of a cigarette every time that urge strikes.

92.   Think of the health implications of quitting smoking. Once you stop, your blood pressure levels are reduced within 20 minutes. After 24 hours, the carbon monoxide levels in your body revert to normal. After about a month, the chance of having a heart attack or stroke decreases, and your lungs will start to function at a better level. All of this is the perfect reason to quit.

93.   Soon after your quit date, head to the dentist for a full teeth cleaning. This will rid yourself of the visual reminders of your time as a smoker. Having bright clean teeth and fresh breath is a concrete item that you can look to when you want a cigarette. When you feel the urge, go take a smile in the mirror and remember what your teeth looked like before. The urge should take a hike!

94.   To increase your chances of being successful in your efforts to quit smoking, consider writing out a list of pros and cons of quitting. When you go through the tactile experience and physical actions of writing, your psychological perspective is often shifted in the process. When you think about your list, it can make your motivation stronger, and keep your focus on the benefits of staying smoke free.

95.   Deal with nicotine withdrawal. Once you quit smoking, nicotine withdrawal can make you anxious, frustrated, or depressed. It's all too easy to revert to your old habit. Nicotine replacement therapy can really help to relieve these symptoms. Whether it's in the form of gum, a patch, or a lozenge, using one of these will probably double your chances of succeeding.

96.   If you're trying to quit smoking, try quitting cold turkey. This method is the easiest in the long run. While this may seem a lot more difficult when you are starting out, it is much easier than stringing your self along. Be honest with your self and commit to the quit and you will be off cigarettes fairly easily.

97.   Make sure you have the right attitude. You can not take quitting as a deprivation. Instead, think of this process as a favor that you are doing for yourself. By quitting you are helping your body and

making a healthier change that will in turn lead to a healthier happier you!

98. Help the symptoms of nicotine withdrawal. If you decide not to use a product that contains nicotine, such as a patch, gum or lozenges, think about asking your doctor about a prescription medication. Certain pills can help to reduce cravings by affecting the chemicals that your brain produces, lessening the symptoms. There are also certain medications that will make a cigarette taste nasty if you decide to smoke.

99. When you are trying to quit smoking, write a list of all of the reasons why you want to stop. Carry that list with you at all times. One of the best place to carry this list is where you used to carry your cigarettes. Whenever you catch yourself reaching for your pack of smokes, pull out the list, instead, and read why you want to break the habit.

100. Take up exercise to help you quit smoking. Exercising is wonderful for both your body and mind. It can help you to focus on the positive things in life, and keep you from thinking about that cigarette that you so dearly want. It is also a wonderful way to meet healthy people. When you're around healthy people, it might just make you want to stay healthy too.

101.   As soon as you decide to quit smoking, tell all of your family and friends. Not only will this help you to build a good support group, but it will also encourage you to stick to your goal. You might even inspire one of your loved ones to quit with you.

102.   When you're ready to quit smoking, and have a plan in place to do so, set a firm date after which you won't smoke anymore. Prepare for the date, and make a big deal out of it. Think of it as the day when you regain control of your life, and make it a joyous occasion.

103.   Make a plan on how to deal with stressful moments. A lot of smokers are accustomed to having a cigarette when encountering a stressful moment. You're less likely to give in to this temptation if you put a plan in place for dealing with stress. Keep a back-up plan handy in case plan A doesn't work out.

104.   Choose the date that you will quit and write it on the calendar. After you've done this, tell your friends and family. Choosing your quit date makes your goal more specific and real so that you're more likely to take action towards it. It's harder to change your mind once you've made a commitment, and

other people can help support you if they know about your quit date.

105.   Try to remember that the mind set is everything. You need to always stay positive as you regard your smoking cessation. Think of all the help and aid you are bringing to your body and how much healthier you are going to be because you have taken this vital step in your life.

106.   If you are about to give up smoking, you need to be aware that the first seven days after you quit will be the toughest. In the first two days, your body will release toxins, specifically nicotine, which might give you some unpleasant feelings. The cravings you experience after that will be predominantly psychological. These symptoms aren't easy to deal with, but are nowhere near as bad as the initial nicotine withdrawal.

107.   To make quitting smoking seem more straightforward, put the negatives of your smoking habit into numbers. For example, figure out how often you smoke, how many cigarettes you smoke a day and how much it costs you to smoke that much on a daily, monthly and yearly basis. Every time you cut back a little, you'll know exactly how much you've progressed.

108.   Stock your refrigerator with fruit juice before quitting. Nicotine releases sugar into your bloodstream, so when you quit you may have massive sugar cravings for a few days. Drinking juice is a healthy way to relieve these cravings. However, if you're diabetic this solution can be dangerous for you, so you should talk to your doctor about safe ways for you to manage sugar cravings.

109.   If you're doing well on your stop smoking journey, don't forget to reward yourself. Treat yourself to a nice massage, a pedicure, or a special new outfit when you've cut back, and then something else when you've stopped entirely. You need to have rewards like this to look forward to, as they can help to keep you motivated.

110.   When aiming to kick the smoking habit for good, you should always believe that you can do it. Think about all the incredible things you have accomplished in your life so far. This will help you realize you have the strength to overcome this addiction. Having faith in yourself is not only important for quitting smoking, but it's also important for overall success in your life.

111.   Using some type of nicotine replacement is a good way to slowly ease your addiction to smoking

when you're trying to quit. Nicotine replacements come in many forms, including lozenges, gum, and patches that can be worn on the body. These products give your body a small dose of nicotine, which eases cravings for using tobacco products.

112.   Commit yourself totally to your decision to quit smoking. If you are determined to quit smoking then put your whole soul into the effort. Announce to family and close friends that you are quitting and need support. Write down your specific goals and make them as detailed as you can. Also write down your individual reasons for quitting. Post both lists where you can easily see them - like the bathroom mirror. Join a support group and attend meetings, whether online or in person. Go all in and make this happen.

113.   When you're trying to stop smoking, allow yourself to get a reward every time you reach a goal. For instance, once a week has gone by without a cigarette, go to a movie. When you make it a whole month without smoking, dine out at a restaurant you really enjoy. Gradually increase the rewards as you finish longer and longer periods without smoking, until it no longer even enters your mind.

114.   Don't assume that a nicotine withdrawal medication has to have nicotine in it. While it is true

that you can find an alternate source of nicotine and reduce your levels of it, you could just try a prescription medication that blocks your need for nicotine. Consult your physician about a medicine that might just kill your cravings.

115.   You can replace your smoking habit with positive coping habits instead. This means really looking inside yourself and examining your habits. If you smoke when you are stressed out, consider how you can diffuse the negative energy instead. Some people find solace in meditative and deep breathing exercises, but you can experiment with a variety of techniques to find one that suits you.

116.   When you have made up your mind that you want to quit smoking, it is important to get some support from others. Let your family, friends, and co-workers know that you are planning on giving up your smoking habit and ask for their support and encouragement. Who knows, some of them may have been successful with breaking the habit and can offer some great advice. With their help and encouragement, it can help you get through the tough days.

117.   If you are trying to kick the smoking habit, counseling may be a good option to try. There are sometimes emotional factors influencing people to

smoke. If that is addressed, the need to smoke may go away. If you feel this might be right for you, talk with your regular physician, and ask for a referral.

118.   When you want to quit smoking, you need to be careful to avoid your triggers. There are some activities that your brain will always associate with smoking. For many people, the trigger is drinking alcohol. For others, it is drinking a cup of coffee. Try reducing your alcohol intake or switching to drinking tea while you are attempting to give up smoking.

119.   In order to quit, you must believe that you can do it. While the physical cravings and withdrawal symptoms of smoking are difficult, your brain is the most important item in your fight. You must be able to work past your cravings and that fight is all mental. Believe that you can do it and you will see success.

120.   While it may be difficult, stay away from other smokers while you are trying to quit, or ask smokers to leave their cigarettes at home for a few weeks when they come to visit. One of the biggest triggers for relapse is simply having the opportunity to smoke, so do not make it easy for yourself to bum one off of anyone.

121.   When you quit smoking, don't forget to drink plenty of water. Drinking water has beneficial effects anyway, but especially when you're trying to stop smoking. It will help flush out the toxins that smoking leaves behind, as well as help satiate your oral fixation, if you have one. If you already drink plenty of water, think about drinking an extra glass the next time you have a craving for a cigarette.

122.   Drink plenty of water when you are quitting cigarettes. The water will help flush the excess toxins from your system. As your body is detoxifying, you need to give the toxins a way out of your body. Keep a bottle of water with you when you are on the go and sip throughout the day.

123.   Remember that smoking cessation is really all about replacing one behavior with another. For most people, it is primarily the physical act of smoking that is the major draw. It signifies "me time" and a break from a hectic schedule or a boring job. Choose ahead of time exactly what behavior you will replace those smoking minutes with, and then do it!

124.   Acupuncture can help you to quit smoking. Acupuncture involves putting some very tiny needles into specific points on your body. It can remove toxins and help to treat unpleasant mental

and physical withdraw symptoms. Be sure to see a reputable and trained professional for this type of treatment, because it can be dangerous if not done correctly.

125.   Try to drink a lot of fruit juice as you begin quitting. The fruit juice will help cleanse your body of all the nicotine that is stored in your system. This will help you better resist cravings that you are bound to get if you do not do this sort of cleanse.

126.   When you are considering quitting smoking, make an appointment to see your physician. Your doctor may have resources for quitting that you may not have. If your doctor thinks that it is appropriate, they may prescribe you medication assist with the quit.

127.   It is extremely important that you talk to a doctor prior to quitting smoking. This person can provide you some advice on your best methods of quitting. In addition, he or she can provide you some additional support on your journey. Both of these things greatly increase your chances of quitting for good.

128.   It is important to realize that although cold turkey may work for one person, it may not work for you. People think that they can quit smoking on

their own and only end up going back because they tried too much, too fast. You may require an aid for quitting, such as a nicotine patch.

129.   When you decide to go out with your family or your friends, try to go to places where you cannot smoke. This will prevent you from taking puffs. Try going to a restaurant or going out to a movie. This is a wonderful way to curve your urges, and it is fairly easy. Just make it inconvenient to smoke.

130.   It is okay to use a nicotine replacement during the beginning stage of your smoking cessation program. Nicotine is highly addictive, and the withdrawal symptoms can be extremely unpleasant. Nicotine gum or lozenges can prevent you from feeling short-tempered, moody and irritable and can be the difference between success and failure.

131.   When planning on quitting smoking, make sure not to let the fear of failure impact the process. Most former smokers had to try more than once before succeeding at kicking their nicotine habits. When you quit, try to stick to abstinence for as long as possible. When you do give into a cigarette, try to quit again immediately after. Quit for longer and longer periods of time each time. One time it will stick, so just be patient.

132.   You need to be clear and committed at every stage of the quitting process. That means setting a firm date at which you want to be done smoking altogether. Use that date to determine smaller goals like when you want to cut back more, and stick to every date without exception.

133.   When you are trying to quit smoking, sometimes you have to change other habits which trigger your desire for a puff. Instead of that cup of coffee or that alcoholic drink, have a glass of juice or water. Many people still have an urge to have a smoke after finishing a meal. After a meal, take a walk. Not only will it help take your mind off having a smoke, it will also help keep off the weight that is commonly associated with giving up smoking.

134.   Keep your motivation for quitting on your mind all the time. You may find it helpful to write inspirational quotes in your planner, or wear a piece of jewelry that reminds you of your struggle. Either way, you may find this visual reminder handy in the face of temptation and craving later.

135.   When you are trying to quit smoking, use the method that works best for you. Some people have more success by quitting gradually, while others do better by quitting cold turkey. Try one method, and

if it does not work for you, switch to the other method to see if it gives you better results.

136.   Clean your house and car when you quit smoking. Don't spend time in any environment where you look at the surroundings and equate them with smoking. Dispose of butts and ashtrays and clean anything with the smell of cigarettes. Your fresh environment should reflect a healthier, cleaner you, and some rigorous housecleaning might just let you power through a craving.

137.   Try some vigorous exercise. Quitting smoking will help improve your lung capacity, making exercise much easier. Keeping active will help you keep from gaining weight too. The endorphins can help take a bit of the edge off the withdrawal symptoms, although their effect cannot compare to that of nicotine.

138.   Do not try to start smoking without first developing a plan. Your life has probably been ruled by cigarettes for quite some time. A life without cigarettes will require adjustments in your life. Deciding what you are going to do about cravings, avoiding triggers, and setting your quit date are all essential components of a successful plan for quitting.

139. Quit smoking to live a healthier life and spend more time with the people you love. Follow the great advice in the following article for ideas on how to quit smoking.

140. Take up exercise to help you quit smoking. Exercising is wonderful for both your body and mind. It can help you to focus on the positive things in life, and keep you from thinking about that cigarette that you so dearly want. It is also a wonderful way to meet healthy people. When you're around healthy people, it might just make you want to stay healthy too.

141. Try to avoid alcohol if you're trying to quit smoking. Alcohol and cigarettes are naturally complimentary to each other. In addition, alcohol lowers your mental focus, meaning you are more likely to give in to temptation or peer pressure. If you avoid alcohol, you're more likely to stay clear of mind. This might just mean that quitting becomes a bit easier.

142. In addition to quitting smoking, you should also cut back on foods and drinks that trigger nicotine cravings. For example, you will be more vulnerable to your nicotine addiction when you drink alcohol. If you regularly drink coffee when you smoke, then

you should cut back on that too to reduce craving-inducing associations.

143.   Blow off some steam to keep yourself from blowing smoke. One of the most effective ways for you to work through nicotine cravings is to exercise. As an added bonus, you will feel the effects of your improving health more readily if you subsidize quitting smoking with a more rigorous exercise routine.

144.   The best advice you can get for quitting smoking is just to stop. Stopping is the only way to start the quitting process. Stop yourself, immediately, and never look back. It may seem quite difficult to do it this way. It has been proven to be effective, as time goes by.

145.   Receiving support from friends and family members can go a long way in helping you to quit smoking. It's especially important to remind them that getting over an addiction can cause mood swings and irritability. If people close to you are understanding of the situation, it will make relapsing that much easier to avoid.

146.   Find an online forum for quitters. This can provide you with a great amount of support and motivation, while still allowing you to remain

anonymous. Online forums can be found everywhere, and you can typically join for free. They will help you to network with individuals all over the world, and you never know what kind of great stop smoking advice you might hear.

147.   Have alternate coping mechanisms in place to deal with the stress that you used handle by smoking before you attempt to quit. Avoid as many stressful situations as possible in the early stages of your attempt to quit. Soothing music, yoga and massage can help you deal with any stress you do encounter.

148.   It can be easier to quit smoking if you are able to articulate exactly why you want to quit. Try writing down a list of all of the reasons that you should quit smoking. This can include the benefits you will experience, people in your life, or any reasons at all that are important to you.

149.   Keep your motivation for quitting on your mind all the time. This could involve you gluing motivational posters and messages to the walls at your work office, or wearing an item of jewelry that symbolizes your intentions to quit. Whatever method you choose, this type of visual reminder may help you ward off craving and temptation.

150. To stay true to your plan to quit smoking, make up motivational note cards to read whenever you get a craving. Keep these cards on your fridge, in your car, in your purse or wallet and even in a drawer at work. Any time a craving strikes, read and repeat the message on the card like a mantra to refocus your efforts.

151. You should make sure you have an appropriate reward system in place for such a difficult task. You will want to reward yourself for at least the first three days of quitting and the first two weeks. After that, monthly milestones are worth a celebration until you hit the annual mark. You can choose your reward based on the time elapsed as well, making success that much sweeter.

152. If you feel like you need a cigarette immediately, then try breathing exercises to calm the craving. This gives you some time to think about the reason you quit. Furthermore, deep breathing increases oxygen intake and encourages you to feel refreshed. Breathing exercises are simple enough to be done anywhere, at any time.

153. To help you quit smoking, you should go to use a stop smoking aide. There are many aides available on the market which you can purchase at your local pharmacy. These aides can help relax your cravings

while you are going through the quitting process. With the use of help, more than likely you will continue to smoke.

154.   Consider keeping a journal of the smoking habits you have developed. Try to figure out when you are most tempted to smoke, so that you can make an appropriate plan to quit. It will be easier to resist your cravings when you prepare yourself ahead of time to do so.

155.   To help you quit smoking, just think of all the health risks associated with this habit. There are so many awful diseases you can get from smoking, such as lung disease, emphysema and all types of cancer. So if you want to get healthy and not be sick all the time, think of the bad things that can occur if you continue to smoke.

156.   Remember that your attitude is everything. When you are beginning to feel down, you need to try to make yourself proud that you are quitting. Smoking is bad for you and each time you conquer the urge to smoke, you should feel proud as you are taking vital steps toward a healthier you.

157.   Stop smoking once and for all by replacing those moments that you enjoy a cigarette with physical exercise. Not only will it be a distraction to

you, but you will also benefit in a huge way by developing a healthier and more attractive body. It may be hard at first due to the effects of nicotine in your system, but start small, with a walk around the block.

158.   Replace your pack of cigarettes with an electronic cigarette. Many former smokers have found success with these devices, which work by vaporizing a liquid that contains nicotine. When the user exhales, the cloud looks just like smoke, but it's actually vapor. Using one of these devices can make it much easier to quit smoking, since it simulates the act so effectively.

159.   Day-by-day is the only way to go about quitting smoking. Take your journey day by day, focusing on the moment instead of the future. A short timeline can help you stay on track instead of worrying about what is coming next. Long term goals will come when you've quit for a while and are better able to handle the daily grind.

160.   Starting an exercise regimen is a great way to support yourself when you're trying to quit smoking. Under the advice of a doctor, ease yourself into the regimen, especially if you've been a heavy smoking for many years. The exercise will help you not only repair some of the damage

smoking has done to your body, but is also a great stress reliever as well.

161.   Tell your relatives that you are quitting, so that they can provide support. Be clear that you need their unwavering support and encouragement, and that anything less could negatively affect your efforts. Remind them that you may have times of frustration and irritability and ask them to bear with you. It is not an easy task to stop smoking and you should make sure your loved one supports you during this process.

162.   As part of your attempt to stop smoking, you will want to discuss it with your physician. Your doctor has access to quit-smoking resources that you don't. In addition, your doctor could prescribe you a medication for quitting if he or she believes that you need to.

163.   See your doctor and ask him to recommend a stop smoking program or medication. Only five percent of people who attempt to stop cold turkey, with no help, succeed in their attempt to quit smoking. You need help to overcome the cravings and withdrawal symptoms that accompany any attempt to quit.

164.   Looking at a picture of smoker's lungs may be all you need to quit smoking. When a person smokes, their lungs turn black after a while and they could end up with lung cancer. As harsh as it may seem, viewing the picture may set off a signal in your brain to quit.

165.   When you're ready to quit smoking, and have a plan in place to do so, set a firm date after which you won't smoke anymore. Prepare for the date, and make a big deal out of it. Think of it as the day when you regain control of your life, and make it a joyous occasion.

166.   It can be easier to quit smoking if you are able to articulate exactly why you want to quit. Try writing down a list of all of the reasons that you should quit smoking. This can include the benefits you will experience, people in your life, or any reasons at all that are important to you.

167.   Remember the following acronym forever: N.O.P.E. It stands for "never one puff, ever." This will be a lifelong motto for you to follow, and it should be your mantra when you are tempted to have "just that one" cigarette. Even if you are out drinking with friends, remember to say N.O.P.E. to that puff!

168. Start moving. Physical activity is a great for reducing nicotine cravings and can ease some of the withdrawal symptoms. When you crave a cigarette, go for a jog instead. Even mild exercise can be helpful, like pulling the weeds in the garden or taking a leisurely stroll. Plus, the extra activity will burn extra calories and help ward off any weight gain as you are quitting smoking.

169. Don't turn back to smoking during a family crisis. Sometimes the most difficult times in our lives, turn into the easiest times to take a bad habit back up. While you might be tempted to do so, try to stay focused on all the reasons that you quit. Talk to a friend or family member about what you're going through or even seek counseling if you need to. Whatever you do, don't reach for that cigarette.

170. If you are thinking about quitting smoking, it is extremely important to have a plan. One of the most important parts of this plan is setting a "quit date." This is the date when you plan to completely stop smoking. Whether you want to quit cold turkey or ease your way into it, having a specific date when you want to be done smoking will help you stay on track.

171. Smoking is an expensive habit in addition to being bad for your health. For some people,

however, even thinking about quitting feels overwhelming. If you want to stop smoking but you don't know what to do, read on. There are lots of techniques to try if you really want to give up.

172.   When you smoke, you sometimes are just obsessed with the feeling of having something in your mouth. This can be replaced with a less dangerous habit such as chewing gum or eating candy. Anytime you feel like smoking, just have a piece of hard candy or chew a stick of gum.

173.   Don't rush into quitting. Take it day-by-day. Focus on giving up cigarettes for the day rather than for the rest of your life. Reaching your goal one day at a time is easier to deal with mentally and physically. Once you are comfortable with the level of commitment you have towards quitting, you can set long term goals.

174.   Take up exercise to help you quit smoking. Exercising is wonderful for both your body and mind. It can help you to focus on the positive things in life, and keep you from thinking about that cigarette that you so dearly want. It is also a wonderful way to meet healthy people. When you're around healthy people, it might just make you want to stay healthy too.

175. Keep a cold glass or bottle of ice water nearby at all times. When you get a craving for a cigarette, take a sip of water--even if this means you hardly put the bottle down at first. This gives you something to do with your hands and mouth, and it can be a useful way to prevent snacking, too.

176. Quit smoking to make exercise easier. Smoking makes it difficult to breathe, meaning that you aren't getting healthy levels of oxygen to your muscles and organs. This makes exercising much more difficult, which can lead to a life filled with ailments. When you quit, your lung capacity will soon improve, making that daily exercise goal, an easier one to achieve.

177. When quitting smoking, you must learn to manage your stress. Once smoking is no longer an option, turn to healthier outlets such as massage therapy, long walks in your favorite park, listening to relaxing music, or meditation. Find something you can do that provides near-instant gratification so that you'll be less tempted to turn to smoking when things get tough.

178. Remember that false starts are common when people try to quit smoking. Even if you've tried and failed to quit before, you should always keep trying. Ultimately, any reduction in your smoking habit is

good for you, so as long as you are trying to quit you are improving your life and health.

179.   To stay motivated to quit cigarettes for good, use the money you save to reward yourself. Figure out how much money you will save by quitting in advance, and put the money you would spend on cigarettes into a special place. Every time you reach a minor goal, use that money to reward yourself with something nice.

180.   Take the time to really sit down and think about how quitting smoking will improve your life. This is especially effective if you already have serious health conditions that smoking can exacerbate, like asthma or diabetes. If your family has a predisposition for cancer, then it can also be very powerful for you to acknowledge that quitting now could actually save your life.

181.   Don't allow yourself "just one puff". The mind can sometimes play tricks on you, especially when you're trying to give up a habit that you have had for years. Don't allow yourself to give in to the idea that just one cigarette won't hurt. It will hurt, and it might just keep you from being able to quit at all.

182.   Find an online forum for quitters. This can provide you with a great amount of support and

motivation, while still allowing you to remain anonymous. Online forums can be found everywhere, and you can typically join for free. They will help you to network with individuals all over the world, and you never know what kind of great stop smoking advice you might hear.

183.   Be open about your intention to quit. Let your friends, family and coworkers know that you are going to do it and when your date is. Current smokers will likely be considerate enough to stop smoking around you at that time. You'll also find out who is supportive and who is critical of your habit. Finding support and sources of encouragement might make a future quitting attempt successful, if this one is not the one.

184.   Master stress management. Aside from nicotine withdrawal and simple habit, a primary reason you might start smoking again is stress. If you can't avoid all stress during the first few weeks after quitting, do whatever it takes to manage your stress in another way than having a cigarette. Get a massage or try a yoga class. Find something new and healthy to replace what you're giving up.

185.   Before beginning to quit, talk with your doctor about your intentions. Your doctor can advise you on the best methods to quit, and if need be, can

provide you with prescription drugs to aid your quitting. Also, your doctor can be an important sounding board throughout your entire quitting experience.

186.   Write down a journal of every time you have a cigarette and what your reasons were for having one. This journal will help you to find out what your smoking triggers are. For some it may be the first morning cigarette, or the need to smoke after a meal. For others, it may be stress. Determining your triggers will help you to figure out a way to fight them.

187.   To become more successful with quitting smoking, try writing the cons and pros of quitting. Just by creating the list, you'll perk up your mood. When you think about your list, it can make your motivation stronger, and keep your focus on the benefits of staying smoke free.

188.   When you feel an urge to smoke and can't resist, at least put it off till later. Tell yourself you need to go for a walk first, or maybe that you need to drink a glass of water first. This break between the craving and its fulfillment may enable to not smoke that cigarette after all. If you do end up smoking a cigarette, at least you will have smoked one less cigarette that day.

189.   Acupuncture can help you to quit smoking. Acupuncture involves putting some very tiny needles into specific points on your body. It can remove toxins and help to treat unpleasant mental and physical withdraw symptoms. Be sure to see a reputable and trained professional for this type of treatment, because it can be dangerous if not done correctly.

190.   Get your loved ones to support you in your decision of kicking your bad smoking habit. Also, make sure that they know not to be judgmental and are as optimistic as possible to improve your chance for success. So, let people around you know that you're going to quit smoking and that your mood is going to change because of this. Quitting smoking is a difficult process, and getting the support of your friends and family is critical.

191.   It is extremely important that you talk to a doctor prior to quitting smoking. This person can provide you some advice on your best methods of quitting. In addition, he or she can provide you some additional support on your journey. Both of these things greatly increase your chances of quitting for good.

192.   Take the money that you would usually throw away on your cigarettes and spend it on yourself on something that you really want. This is sort of like a reward for your hard work. Treat yourself to an expensive coat, a nice jacket or even that pair of shoes that you have been eying.

193.   Find another way to relax. Nicotine is a relaxant, so you need to find a substitute to lessen your stress. A massage or yoga is a really great way of relaxing, or you could try a warm bath, or listening to your favorite music. Whenever possible, try to stay away from anything stressful during the initial couple of weeks when you stop smoking.

194.   Create a plan to reward yourself each time you reach a milestone in your quitting efforts. Come up with a worthwhile reward for every set amount of days, weeks or months you go without smoking. For motivational reasons, make sure you have your reward chart somewhere it is easily seen by you. It might provide inspiration and motivation during difficult times.

195.   When trying to quit smoking, set a goal. Tell yourself that you want to quit by a certain date and that if you are successful, you will reward yourself with something you have been wanting. You can use the money you saved by not smoking to buy

this treat! This will give you the motivation you need.

196. Having a fixed date for when you want to be done with smoking can give you something to focus on. Deadlines often make it easier to achieve a task, and quitting smoking is no different. If you tell yourself that you must quit by a certain date, you will make a greater effort to do so.

197. When you are trying to quit smoking, use the method that works best for you. Some people have more success by quitting gradually, while others do better by quitting cold turkey. Try one method, and if it does not work for you, switch to the other method to see if it gives you better results.

198. Rid your home of anything cigarette related. Once you decide to quit smoking, get rid of any evidence. Throw away ashtrays, lighters, matches etc. Wash your clothes and clean the house from top to bottom. The last thing you need is a scent of cigarettes that might lure you back in to the habit.

199. Clean your house and car when you quit smoking. Don't spend time in any environment where you look at the surroundings and equate them with smoking. Dispose of butts and ashtrays and clean anything with the smell of cigarettes.

Your fresh environment should reflect a healthier, cleaner you, and some rigorous housecleaning might just let you power through a craving.

200.   Thinking about the impacts that smoking has on your family can serve as a serious motivator to stop smoking. Statistics say that one in five deaths in America alone are tied to smoking cigarettes. Don't let yourself be one of the ones who dies from smoking. Quit today for better health.

201.   Consult your doctor about quitting. Your doctor can prescribe smoking cessation aids such as nicotine gum or nicotine patches. In addition, your doctor may know some strategies for controlling cravings that you don't know. He can help you create a plan to stop smoking as well as monitoring your health while you work on quitting.

202.   If the fear of gaining weight is the only thing holding you back from quitting, you should know that gaining weight is not inevitable. Many former smokers never gain any weight when they quit. That said, gaining a few pounds is still far healthier than continuing to smoke. With a bit of exercise and mindful snacking, this fear should play no part in keeping you from quitting.

203.   If you're trying to quit smoking, try quitting cold turkey. This method is the easiest in the long run. While this may seem a lot more difficult when you are starting out, it is much easier than stringing your self along. Be honest with your self and commit to the quit and you will be off cigarettes fairly easily.

204.   Set a series of intermediate goals as part of your program to stop smoking. As you achieve each goal, reward yourself. On your one week anniversary you could visit a movie, for example. When you go an entire month, go to a fancy restaurant you don't normally go to. Build up the rewards until you are completely free of cigarettes.

205.   Remember that false starts are common when people try to quit smoking. Even if you've tried and failed to quit before, you should always keep trying. Ultimately, any reduction in your smoking habit is good for you, so as long as you are trying to quit you are improving your life and health.

206.   Keeping a positive attitude can be the extra motivation to stop smoking. Think about the improvement to your life you will have. Consider that your teeth are going to be brighter and cleaner, your breath and clothes will smell better, and your home is going to be full of freshness and cleanliness. If the side effects of smoking are not

enough to motivate you, think about the many different benefits.

207.   When you are trying to quit smoking, sometimes you have to change other habits which trigger your desire for a puff. Instead of that cup of coffee or that alcoholic drink, have a glass of juice or water. Many people still have an urge to have a smoke after finishing a meal. After a meal, take a walk. Not only will it help take your mind off having a smoke, it will also help keep off the weight that is commonly associated with giving up smoking.

208.   When you are trying to quit smoking, use the method that works best for you. Some people have more success by quitting gradually, while others do better by quitting cold turkey. Try one method, and if it does not work for you, switch to the other method to see if it gives you better results.

209.   To clarify why it is so important for you to quit, ask the people you love to tell you how they think smoking has affected you. Just be prepared to hear unpleasant comments about how your car or clothes smell or more emotional confessions like how your kids worry about your health.

210.   If you want to quit smoking, stop buying cigarettes. It kind of goes without saying that if you

don't have cigarettes on you, it will be much more difficult to smoke. Throw away any cigarettes that are currently in your possession and make a pact with yourself not to buy any more.

211.   Don't let yourself indulge even a little bit. It is easy to tell yourself that one cigarette will be fine, but it may undo all of your dedication and hard work, and it really isn't worth it in the long run. Remember that even one cigarette can restart the mental addiction.

212.   When you have made up your mind that you want to quit smoking, it is important to get some support from others. Let your family, friends, and co-workers know that you are planning on giving up your smoking habit and ask for their support and encouragement. Who knows, some of them may have been successful with breaking the habit and can offer some great advice. With their help and encouragement, it can help you get through the tough days.

213.   If you are pregnant, or plan or becoming that way, then use this as a serious motivation to stop smoking. Statistics say that women who smoke while carrying a child, especially in the first trimester, will cause the infant to have a decreased

body weight. This will in turn affect their health, potentially throughout childhood.

214.   Be mindful of what your habits are. When do you want to smoke the most? Quitting smoking can be a difficult process, so you must be prepared to handle cravings.

215.   When trying to quit smoking, ensure that you're using common sense when it comes to eating. Do not quit smoking and start a diet in the same week. However, eat balanced meals as much as possible. Research shows that vegetables, fruits, as well as low-fat dairy products tend to leave an unwanted taste on your mouth if you're smoking. If you eat these items, it will boost your immune system and help you quit.

216.   Drink plenty of water when you are quitting cigarettes. The water will help flush the excess toxins from your system. As your body is detoxifying, you need to give the toxins a way out of your body. Keep a bottle of water with you when you are on the go and sip throughout the day.

217.   Cut your caffeine intake in half. Somehow, nicotine cuts the effectiveness of caffeine in half, so after quitting, soda and coffee will be doubly effective. Drop your consumption of these so that

you don't cause your anxiety to become even worse than it already is at this difficult time.

218.   Instead of committing to smoking, make a life commitment to exercise. Gradually, your body will begin to flush out all toxins; you will then begin to notice improved endurance and higher energy levels. As you strengthen your body through exercise, you will be much less likely to ruin those efforts by sneaking a cigarette.

219.   You do not have to stay addicted to cigarettes, the choice is yours.

220.   If you want to quit smoking, the word for you is "No". Every time you're tempted you have to disallow yourself the ability to say "Yes" to a cigarette. If your only answer is "No" you'll find that you can't cave in to a craving. No cigarettes, no "Maybe", leads to no smoking!

221.   If you're doing well on your stop smoking journey, don't forget to reward yourself. Treat yourself to a nice massage, a pedicure, or a special new outfit when you've cut back, and then something else when you've stopped entirely. You need to have rewards like this to look forward to, as they can help to keep you motivated.

222.   Start up some type of exercise, in order to keep your mind busy, and stay away from cigarettes. Movement of any kind is also an effective tool for stress relief. If you do not exercise normally, you can start by taking short walks outside daily. Don't exercise without consulting your physician about what are safe and appropriate exercises for you.

223.   Improve your chances of successfully quitting by sharing your plan to quit with supportive loved ones and friends. The encouragement you receive can provide extra motivation during rough patches, and telling people about quitting will help you stay more accountable. Have a few people on stand-by whom you can call for distraction whenever you get a craving.

224.   Avoid triggering that make you want to smoke. Alcohol is a trigger for many, so when you are quitting, try to drink less. If coffee is your trigger, for a couple of weeks drink tea instead. If you like to smoke after eating a meal, do something else rather like taking a walk or brushing your teeth.

225.   If you want to quit smoking, don't do it. Quitting smoking are two words that imply losing something, making it a grieving process. Instead, psychologically embrace tobacco freedom. Don't think about how you would make anyone else

happy, but what would make you happy if you were free from cigarettes. What could you do with that money and time?

226.   If you are looking for a quick pick me up like a cigarette gives you, try to have a glass of juice instead. This will help you cut down on the amount of cigarettes you have each day, and give you something that is healthy to replace smoking with.

227.   Remember that the hardest part of quitting is usually those first couple of days. Mentally prepare yourself to tough it out for just the first two days, and then just the first week, and you will probably be in good shape after that. Your body will be doing a good amount of detoxifying in those first few days and if you can make it through that stage, you can make it through anything.

228.   Be open about your intention to quit. Let your friends, family and coworkers know that you are going to do it and when your date is. Current smokers will likely be considerate enough to stop smoking around you at that time. You'll also find out who is supportive and who is critical of your habit. Finding support and sources of encouragement might make a future quitting attempt successful, if this one is not the one.

229.   If you want to quit smoking, stop buying cigarettes. It kind of goes without saying that if you don't have cigarettes on you, it will be much more difficult to smoke. Throw away any cigarettes that are currently in your possession and make a pact with yourself not to buy any more.

230.   Don't use weight gain as an excuse to continue smoking. While it is true that some individuals gain weight when they quit, it doesn't mean that you will. Make healthy eating choices when you're feeling hungry because you aren't smoking and the weight won't pile on. Even if you do gain a few pounds, remember that it is much healthier than continuing to smoke.

231.   If you do not want to use nicotine replacement therapy to help you quit smoking, consider asking your doctor for a prescription. There are medications that can alter your brain chemistry and reduce your nicotine cravings. Taking one of these prescriptions may be just the aid you need to get you over the hump.

232.   Put the cash you would have spent on smoking in a jar and watch it add up! When you've reached a good amount of cash, treat yourself to something nice. Seeing all of that money pile up might just help you to realize how much you were wasting on

cigarettes. Being able to treat yourself to something special will become it's own motivator too.

233.   To assist in your quest to ban smoking from your life, seek out another smoker who is attempting to quit, and provide each other some support. The only people who can truly understand what you're going through are the ones who are going through the exact same situation you are in. Share tips with each other and give positive words to each other, whenever one of you feels like giving in to temptation. Trying to quit with someone else is much more effective than trying to quit on your own.

234.   Remember when you begin quitting that the law of addiction is absolutely a part of the equation. This "law" basically emphasizes that giving a drug of choice to an addicted person within the detoxification period will immediately reinstate an addiction. This can be be a worse addiction than it was originally, making smoking within the first 72 hours not worth it!

235.   By using this information, and following the provided tips, you can be successful and reach your goal of being cigarette free.

236.   To increase your chances of being successful in your efforts to quit smoking, consider writing out a list of pros and cons of quitting. Writing something down can change your whole mental outlook. You'll be able to use the list as motivation whenever you need it, helping to focus you on your goals.

237.   If you're trying to quit smoking, try chewing gum instead. Often times when you try to leave a bad habit behind, you must replace it with a more positive one. Chewing gum allows you to use your mouth and jaw in some of the same ways that smoking does. It is a healthy way to keep yourself busy while you're working toward quitting.

238.   Help the symptoms of nicotine withdrawal. If you decide not to use a product that contains nicotine, such as a patch, gum or lozenges, think about asking your doctor about a prescription medication. Certain pills can help to reduce cravings by affecting the chemicals that your brain produces, lessening the symptoms. There are also certain medications that will make a cigarette taste nasty if you decide to smoke.

239.   Try to create a list of reasons why you are quitting. Keep it handy. This list will serve as a reminder of all the things that you are getting by quitting in the long run. Every time you feel the

urge to smoke, try to take a good long look at your list and it will help you stick to your plan.

240.   Try to encourage friends and family to support your decision to stop smoking. Be clear that you need their unwavering support and encouragement, and that anything less could negatively affect your efforts. Let them know that you'll be moody at the beginning, since your thinking won't be as clear. Quitting is one of the most difficult things a smoker may have to go through in their life and gaining the support of your loved ones is imperative to your success.

241.   Talk to your doctor about quitting smoking. Your physician may have resources available to help you quit that you do not have access to. Additionally, your doctor might feel that you would benefit from using a prescription drug therapy method to help you quit.

242.   Cravings seem to come most often when an individual is feeling stressed. To keep yourself from falling victim to this, find a healthy alternative for stress relief. Adopt healthier habits and hobbies such as working out, taking long walks, or listening to music and dancing. When you've got downtime, distract yourself with friends, books and games, so you don't think of smoking.

243.   If you have very strong associations between smoking and drinking coffee or smoking while you're drinking, you may need to avoid these triggers for a while. Once you feel comfortable enough in your ability to stay away from cigarettes, you can slowly bring back that morning cup of joe or happy hour with your friends.

244.   It is okay to use a nicotine replacement during the beginning stage of your smoking cessation program. Nicotine is highly addictive, and the withdrawal symptoms can be extremely unpleasant. Nicotine gum or lozenges can prevent you from feeling short-tempered, moody and irritable and can be the difference between success and failure.

245.   Do some exercise to assist your goals of eliminating smoking from your life. Exercise just doesn't go with smoking. Regular exercise can eliminate your stress, and it assists your body in eliminating the bad effects that smoking causes. If you're new to exercising, start out slow by just walking once or twice a day. Eventually, you can build up to more rigorous exercise for around thirty minutes a day three or four times per week. As always, talk to your doctor prior to starting an exercise routine.

246.   The best way to quit for good is to quit for the right reasons. You should not quit for the people around you. You should quit for yourself. You should make a decision that you want to live a happier, healthier lifestyle and stick to it. This is the best way to ensure success.

247.   Enlist your friends and family to support you with your decision to stop smoking. Those closest to you can be a real help in keeping you on track and smoke-free. Inform everyone of your intentions to quit smoking before your quit date, and let them know specifically how they can be of best help to you.

248.   Master stress management. Aside from nicotine withdrawal and simple habit, a primary reason you might start smoking again is stress. If you can't avoid all stress during the first few weeks after quitting, do whatever it takes to manage your stress in another way than having a cigarette. Get a massage or try a yoga class. Find something new and healthy to replace what you're giving up.

249.   Don't give up if you slip up. Anytime someone tries to give something up that they have been doing for years, there will likely be a struggle. When that struggle exists, slip ups often happen. If you do slip up, get right back on track and try again. The

worst thing you can do is turn a slip up into an excuse to keep smoking, so don't do it.

250.	Stay away from the kind of situations where you would be tempted to smoke. If you associate smoking with drinking a cup of coffee in the morning or attending happy hour when the workday is done, you will probably need to adjust your routine. If you don't go to happy hour, you may be able to avoid the cravings.

251.	Before you begin the process of quitting your nicotine habit for good, take the time to make a specific plan of action. Merely thinking that you can muster up the willpower when needed is a poor way to approach this very addictive habit. Write down a list of things that you will do instead of reaching for that cigarette. This can include going for a walk, calling a friend, making a fresh fruit smoothie, or any number of diversions.

252.	Help the symptoms of nicotine withdrawal. If you decide not to use a product that contains nicotine, such as a patch, gum or lozenges, think about asking your doctor about a prescription medication. Certain pills can help to reduce cravings by affecting the chemicals that your brain produces, lessening the symptoms. There are also certain medications that will make a cigarette taste nasty if you decide to smoke.

253.   Make sure you do not feel as if you have to give up any aspect of your life because you are quitting smoking. Anything that you do you can still do as an ex-smoker. Who knows, you may even be able to do your favorite things a little bit better.

254.   In order to succeed with your goal of quitting smoking, it's important that you write down the benefits that are derived from quitting smoking. Some examples include living a longer life, feeling great, smelling better, saving money, etc. Lots of benefits are gained from eliminating smoking from your life. Writing them down can help to keep you motivated to succeed.

255.   Receiving support from friends and family members can go a long way in helping you to quit smoking. It's especially important to remind them that getting over an addiction can cause mood swings and irritability. If people close to you are understanding of the situation, it will make relapsing that much easier to avoid.

256.   Write down why you're quitting ahead of time and keep that list handy. When that craving hits you, refer to your list for motivation. Understanding

ahead of time why quitting is important to you will help to keep you focused in those moments of weakness, and it might even help to get you back on track if you should slip up.

257.   Do not try to set a day to quit. Instead of trying to make a plan, quit today. This sort of planning nearly never works and it will lead to disappointment. Start quitting right away, rather than trying to create an imaginary timeline for yourself. Take action and you will get where you want to be.

258.   Remember that the hardest part of quitting is usually those first couple of days. Mentally prepare yourself to tough it out for just the first two days, and then just the first week, and you will probably be in good shape after that. Your body will be doing a good amount of detoxifying in those first few days and if you can make it through that stage, you can make it through anything.

259.   Start moving. Physical activity is a great for reducing nicotine cravings and can ease some of the withdrawal symptoms. When you crave a cigarette, go for a jog instead. Even mild exercise can be helpful, like pulling the weeds in the garden or taking a leisurely stroll. Plus, the extra activity will

burn extra calories and help ward off any weight gain as you are quitting smoking.

260.   If you have a friend or loved one who is having a hard time trying to quit, then you should try sharing with them some of the painful truths about smoking. Try to be sincere and understanding as you relate this information so that they understand that you are trying to help them and that you are not trying to attack them.

261.   If you're trying to stop smoking, stay away from situations or places that could tempt you to smoke. If you've always had cigarettes during your happy hour or with your coffee, try changing this type of routine. Drinking coffee on your way to work in the car, or finding a new hangout besides the bar, will give you a chance to minimize familiar triggers and cravings.

262.   Avoid emptying your ashtrays. If you see how many cigarettes you have smoked laying the the ashtray, you will be less likely to smoke any more. This will also leave the unsightly butts and their smell behind. This can be helpful because it will remind of you how bad the smell of smoke is.

263.   If you are trying to quit with the use of crutches such as patches and medication, then you need to

be careful. When you begin taking in these other substances, you are in turn putting yourself at risk of developing a new dangerous addiction. Be careful when you begin your quitting crutches.

264.   Try to remember that the mind set is everything. You need to always stay positive as you regard your smoking cessation. Think of all the help and aid you are bringing to your body and how much healthier you are going to be because you have taken this vital step in your life.

265.   Getting rid of anything that can remind you of smoking is beneficial for anyone trying to kick the habit. Get rid of all the ashtrays and lighters in your home. Clean your carpets, drapes and furniture as well as your linens, towels and clothing to remove the stench of smoke. Doing these things will make it less likely that you will be reminded about smoking and wind up with a cigarette craving.

266.   If you wish to quit smoking cold turkey, get rid of all of the things in your house that remind you of smoking. This means, no more ash trays or cigarette lighters. If you hold onto this stuff, you'll only be reminded of smoking and it might make you want to have a cigarette.

267.   If you have decided to stop smoking, mentally prepare yourself for what's ahead. Try to focus on the fact that you can stop, and that this is not an impossible dream. Set an official "quit date" and even consider adding it to your calendar. By taking such a positive approach, your chances of quitting will increase.

268.   Remember that your attitude is everything. When you are beginning to feel down, you need to try to make yourself proud that you are quitting. Smoking is bad for you and each time you conquer the urge to smoke, you should feel proud as you are taking vital steps toward a healthier you.

269.   Before you begin your plan to stop smoking, create a personalized list of steps you can take to quit. Take time to customize your list as a way to quit smoking more effectively. What works for someone else may not work for you. It's vital that you figure out the ways that work best for you. Making a list for yourself of your own methods will help you reach your goal.

270.   When you are trying to quit smoking, write a list of all of the reasons why you want to stop. Carry that list with you at all times. One of the best place to carry this list is where you used to carry your cigarettes. Whenever you catch yourself reaching

for your pack of smokes, pull out the list, instead, and read why you want to break the habit.

271.   If you want to quit smoking, you need to identify factors that will motivate you to stop. Preventing lung cancer, tooth decay, gum disease and emphysema, or protecting your family are strong motivators. Showing respect for your body and for the gift of life is also a powerful motivating force. Whatever reason you choose, it needs to be enough to prevent you from lighting up again in the future.

272.   Talk to your doctor about prescription medicines. If you want to ease nicotine withdrawal symptoms, consider prescription medications. There are certain medications that affect the chemical balance in your brain and can help reduce cravings. There are also drugs that can reduce bothersome withdrawal symptoms, like inability to concentrate or depression.

273.   Stay away from alcohol or other things that trigger an urge to smoke. Alcohol and coffee are a known trigger for smoking, so stay away from them if possible. Also, smokers tend to light up after eating, so find something else to do, such as washing the dishes or cleaning your teeth.

274.   Tell everyone you know the great news - you're quitting! They will be there for whatever you need and can remind you of your plans to quit. Using a good support system is beneficial when quitting. This greatly increases the chances that you'll succeed, and it'll get you where you want to be.

275.   Blow off some steam to keep yourself from blowing smoke. One of the most effective ways for you to work through nicotine cravings is to exercise. As an added bonus, you will feel the effects of your improving health more readily if you subsidize quitting smoking with a more rigorous exercise routine.

276.   To stay motivated to quit cigarettes for good, use the money you save to reward yourself. Figure out how much money you will save by quitting in advance, and put the money you would spend on cigarettes into a special place. Every time you reach a minor goal, use that money to reward yourself with something nice.

277.   If you want to quit smoking, don't do it. Quitting smoking are two words that imply losing something, making it a grieving process. Instead, psychologically embrace tobacco freedom. Don't think about how you would make anyone else happy, but what would make you happy if you were

free from cigarettes. What could you do with that money and time?

278.   Consider any therapy that can replace nicotine. Smoking itself is kind of disgusting and easy to give up, but the nicotine withdrawal usually proves the nail in the coffin of a quit attempt. Do whatever you can to deal with the withdrawal, from medicine prescriptions to alternatives like the patch, gum or even throat lozenges.

279.   Get support through online forums and support communities. You'll find many different groups which are open to all or focus on a niche. It may be helpful or even cathartic to share quitting frustrations and successes with others who understand your struggle. Other ex-smokers understand your challenges and the emotional problems that sometimes get in the way of quitting smoking.

280.   If you are trying to quit with the use of crutches such as patches and medication, then you need to be careful. When you begin taking in these other substances, you are in turn putting yourself at risk of developing a new dangerous addiction. Be careful when you begin your quitting crutches.

281.   When you are trying to quit smoking, do not attempt to do it overnight. Nicotine addiction is powerful, and it is going to take you some time to wean yourself off of it. You are much more likely to relapse if you quit cold turkey, so take it slow and get it right the first time.

282.   Write out the benefits of quitting smoking to add to your motivation and eliminate cigarettes from your daily routine. Putting something down in writing can alter your entire outlook. This can help you stay motivated, and may make quitting easier.

283.   If you're doing well on your stop smoking journey, don't forget to reward yourself. Treat yourself to a nice massage, a pedicure, or a special new outfit when you've cut back, and then something else when you've stopped entirely. You need to have rewards like this to look forward to, as they can help to keep you motivated.

284.   Keep a cold glass or bottle of ice water nearby at all times. When you get a craving for a cigarette, take a sip of water--even if this means you hardly put the bottle down at first. This gives you something to do with your hands and mouth, and it can be a useful way to prevent snacking, too.

285.   Get into a fitness routine by joining a gym and occupy your smoking time with beneficial exercise. Exercise can go a long way to reducing the stress brought on by nicotine withdrawals. If you don't exercise regularly, try to begin slow by taking walks once or twice daily. Ask your doctor, before you start engaging in any exercise activities.

286.   Be cognizant of routine activities that trigger the desire to have a smoke. For some, it is the first cup of coffee in the morning. For others it may be the end of a meal, or socializing with smoking friends. Whatever your trigger may be, this is the time you must remind yourself that you are quitting because you care enough about yourself that you want to.

287.   Believe it or not, exercise can be the key you need to quitting smoking. Usually, many people smoke because they feel overwhelmed or stressed out. When they feel stressed, they turn to cigarettes for support. Cigarettes can be replaced by exercise. Also, exercise is good for a person's overall health.

288.   Many people find the electronic cigarettes a great way to quit smoking. They do not have as many of the negative effects of normal cigarettes and can be a good way to taper off your smoking from your normal levels to a lesser point, until you are no longer smoking at all.

289.   Commit to quitting. Individuals who are able to successfully quit smoking commit themselves fully. They don't have a back up plan, they don't keep quitting a secret, and they don't tell themselves that they will fail. If you make this type of commitment you will significantly increase your chances of successfully meeting your goal.

290.   The best way to quit smoking is to completely stop. Stopping completely is the only way to really quit. Just try to stop completely and never pick up another cigarette. This method of quitting cigarettes is not the easiest one. It has been shown that this method can be quite effective.

291.   While part of the idea of quitting smoking is to save money, treat yourself to a reward now and again with the money that you haven't spent on cigarettes. These treats give your something to look forward to and serve as a reminder of the things you may not have been able to buy as a smoker.

292.   You should make sure you have an appropriate reward system in place for such a difficult task. You will want to reward yourself for at least the first three days of quitting and the first two weeks. After that, monthly milestones are worth a celebration until you hit the annual mark. You can choose your

reward based on the time elapsed as well, making success that much sweeter.

293.   Many smokers have certain triggers that create the sudden need for a cigarette, such as feeling stressed, ending a meal, or being at a certain location. When you are trying to quit, avoid these triggers if you can. If you can't avoid them, come up with some way to distract yourself from the need to smoke.

294.   Make "NOPE, not one puff, ever" your mantra. You can convince yourself that one cigarette won't hurt, but it may undo a lot of dedication and hard work. Keep in mind what a single puff can do.

295.   Drink lots of cranberry juice the first three days. Any consumption of acidic fruit juices will really take the edge off of the nicotine withdrawal as your internal chemistry slowly accepts the change. Just remember to quit after three days, as the physical nicotine withdrawal will end by then and the juices will just fatten you up after that.

296.   Add exercise to your regular routine if you are trying to smoke. Physical activity can help you to deal with the nicotine cravings you will experience. Exercise can help to lessen these withdrawal symptoms. Get out and walk the dog or dig in your

garden, and you will have an easier time quitting smoking.

297.   You should be honest with yourself when you are looking to quit smoking. Your addiction to tobacco is as real as any other substance addiction. This means that you should seek out emotional and physical support to assist you in quitting cigarettes. Furthermore, this also means that quitting smoking should be all or nothing.

298.   Put a little effort into choosing a quit day. Ideally, set your quit date far enough in the future that you can plan for it, but not so far away that it seems intangible. Do not choose a day that will be busy or stressful, and clearly mark the date on your calendar so that you can prepare for it.

299.   If you're trying to quit smoking, try quitting cold turkey. This method is the easiest in the long run. While this may seem a lot more difficult when you are starting out, it is much easier than stringing your self along. Be honest with your self and commit to the quit and you will be off cigarettes fairly easily.

300.   Consider visiting a hypnotist for help in kicking the habit. If you decide to try hypnosis, make an appointment with a licensed hypnotist. The hypnotist will induce a deep trance, and then repeat

positive affirmations that will lodge themselves in your mind. These affirmations will be in your subconscious, which will aid you on your way to quitting smoking.

301.   Prior to starting to quit smoking, be able to stay committed to quitting for good. Too many people try to quit on a whim and then fail when they are faced with serious obstacles. It is possible for you to maintain a high level of commitment by keeping in mind the reasons why you want to quit.

302.   To cut back on smoking cravings, change the habits that once surrounded smoking. For example, if you always smoked on your breaks then see if you can get your breaks at a different time to make it harder to succumb to those cravings. Likewise, if you always had a cigarette with coffee then switch to a new caffeine fix like tea.

303.   Giving up tobacco will benefit your loved ones, and yourself. Secondhand smoke is very dangerous and causes various types of cancer, as well as many other health conditions. Your family members will spend less time exposed to the dangers of secondhand smoke when you stop smoking. Quitting will improve the health of yourself and your loved ones.

304.   Blow off some steam to keep yourself from blowing smoke. One of the most effective ways for you to work through nicotine cravings is to exercise. As an added bonus, you will feel the effects of your improving health more readily if you subsidize quitting smoking with a more rigorous exercise routine.

305.   Have alternate coping mechanisms in place to deal with the stress that you used handle by smoking before you attempt to quit. Avoid as many stressful situations as possible in the early stages of your attempt to quit. Soothing music, yoga and massage can help you deal with any stress you do encounter.

306.   When you are trying to quit smoking, sometimes you have to change other habits which trigger your desire for a puff. Instead of that cup of coffee or that alcoholic drink, have a glass of juice or water. Many people still have an urge to have a smoke after finishing a meal. After a meal, take a walk. Not only will it help take your mind off having a smoke, it will also help keep off the weight that is commonly associated with giving up smoking.

307.   You should make sure you have an appropriate reward system in place for such a difficult task. You will want to reward yourself for at least the first

three days of quitting and the first two weeks. After that, monthly milestones are worth a celebration until you hit the annual mark. You can choose your reward based on the time elapsed as well, making success that much sweeter.

308.   Avoid situations where you may be strongly tempted to smoke, especially places where alcohol is served. If you find yourself at a party, or bar, or similar place, it may be very tough to keep your determination not to smoke. If you drink alcohol, which lowers inhibitions, it will be much more difficult as well.

309.   When cravings strike, remember that they almost always pass within 10 minutes, so do something to distract yourself. Walk to the water cooler, have a healthy snack, meditate, or call a supportive friend to keep your mind off your craving. You'll be surprised at how quickly it's over, and your delaying tactics can keep you from giving in.

310.   Try to put quitting in a positive light, as it can serve to be very advantageous to your life. You will find it easier to achieve positive results, if you view the choice in that light. Remind yourself of how important your task is, and keep in mind that the positive aspects of quitting outweigh the negative

ones by a long shot. This keeps you on track and makes quitting seem immediately important.

311.   To optimize your chances of success, don't try to quit smoking during a stressful time in your life. This is when your nicotine addiction is strongest, and trying to quit only sets you up for failure. Wait until you feel empowered by other successes - regardless of how large or small - and use that success as a springboard for quitting.

312.   Check with your health department, local clinics, or doctor's office for information about local support groups for those who want to quit smoking. Talking to others who are quitting can provide valuable coping tips, support, and motivation. This may prove especially helpful if your friends and family are not supportive of your desire to quit.

313.   In order to quit, you must believe that you can do it. While the physical cravings and withdrawal symptoms of smoking are difficult, your brain is the most important item in your fight. You must be able to work past your cravings and that fight is all mental. Believe that you can do it and you will see success.

www.ingramcontent.com/pod-product-compliance
Lightning Source LLC
Chambersburg PA
CBHW060751260726
48660CB00002B/566